HEALING
THE HEART

A Story of King David

Harvest of Healing, LLC

Izauh 61®

HARVEST OF HEALING, LLC

Izauh 61®

Publishing assistance by BookCrafters, Parker, Colorado.
www.bookcrafters.net

Isaiah 61:1: The <u>Spirit</u> of the Lord God is on Me, because the Lord has anointed Me to bring good news to the poor. He has sent Me to <u>heal the brokenhearted</u>, to proclaim liberty to the captives and freedom to the prisoners. (HCS) (emphasis added)

TABLE OF CONTENTS

ETYMOLOGY OF KEY WORDS
2 Samuel Chapters 11 and 12
King James Bible

*Note: "Father" does not always direct the attention toward God as being Father. The title father is also reflective of a teacher, one who is in a position of authority that leads or directs.

Abimelech: Father (protector, ruler, paternity, authority, leadership) + king, royalty.

Abner: Father + light or lamp. Father of light (someone who teaches about the light within). (2 Samuel 3:17-39)

Ammonite: Son of my people; beloved of Yahweh.

Bathsheba: Daughter (lineage) + seven (7=completeness, perfection, divine fulfillment). To take an oath.

David: Beloved or loved one; friend.

Eliam: God + nation or people. God's people.

Hittite: Canaanite people; descendant of Heth; person of Hatti. (Slight connection to fear or dread.)

Jedidiah: God's friend; beloved or friend.

Jerubbesheth: To contend or strive; to plead a cause; shame, disgrace, confusion.

Joab: Yahweh is Father; God has/is the fatherly role.

Laish: Lion, a strong, lion-like figure; to knead, gentle.

Nathan: To give; he gave; gift.

Paltiel: God is my deliverance; to escape; to bring into security.

Rabbah: Great; many; abundant; great city.

Solomon: Peace, wholeness; man of peace.

Thebez: Brightness or splendor; mud, mire, clay. (I interpret the mud, mire, clay as: challenged to move forward in life; actions that take extra effort.)

Uriah: Light, flame or fire; divine presence, enlightenment or favor.

INTRODUCTION

Is it possible that physical ailments, illness or disease could be rooted in active church attendance? A form of declining health that comes before the diagnosis of high cholesterol, heart attack or other life-altering disease that is ever-present today. As you move through the following chapters and follow along with the Scriptures referenced, a deep root to disease that has been buried under the soil of our flesh will be exposed.

Is every answer or remedy for failing health contained in the information provided herein? Absolutely not. As new information comes to light, there will be a measure of time required to iron out any wrinkles and put manicured labels on what I attempt to explain. Once again, buckle up for the ride as we explore the depths of the Story of King David.

<u>Psalm 103:1-7</u>: My soul praise Yahweh, and all that is within me, praise His holy name. My soul, praise the Lord and do not forget all His benefits. He forgives all your sin; He heals all your diseases. He redeems your life from the Pit; He crowns you with faithful love and compassion. He satisfies you with goodness; your youth is renewed like the eagle. The Lord executes acts of righteousness and justice for all the oppressed. He revealed His ways to Moses, His deeds to the people of Israel. (HCS)

OVERVIEW

The Heart Breaks

Anyone who has experienced periods of unexplained fatigue, lack of interest, feeling tired yet can't seem to sleep to the point of being rested, or happiness seems impossible to attain, could be suffering from a broken heart. The broken heart is not necessarily rooted in a physical malfunction, as of yet, but a lack of sufficient Heavenly Gases (chemical elements) that builds a foundation for chronic health related issues. It becomes a challenge to be rested or have sufficient strength to get through the day and being joyful is simply out of the ballpark. These symptoms, often grouped with a classification of emotional, may need a closer look. The onset of a heart condition or other organ malfunction could be in the making. The lack of gases is rooted in several causes that reach back through the sands of time to none other than King David.

Today, the broken heart a person experiences can be genetic, can wax and wane throughout a person's life or can delay or intensify its symptoms over a period of years. Nonetheless, a broken heart is an issue that can be locked in place within the depths of the cells and DNA structure that eventually leads to damaged chromosomes. Over an extended period, possibly generations, this broken heart will open the door for chronic conditions and disease.

Using a panoramic view of the story of King David sheds light upon the use of the term Husband in Scripture. The role of the cosmic Husband is played by Uriah, who dies in battle. Today, when the title husband is present, we think of the male figure within a relationship that is joined by some type of commitment or ceremony. In Scripture, the term Husband is speaking of a signaling process that comes from the Heavens and interacts with the human body, particularly the brain and spine. A more in-depth study on Husband will be had in the future.

Scripture paints the picture of how the loss of, we'll call it the cosmic Husband experience, can influence the physical body to the point the body begins to malfunction, starting with the brain. This breakdown of cosmic union between the electro-magnetic field that exists in the Heavens, and the human brain (and animals as well; Psalm 150:6) has been a progressive issue for many years.

In Chapter 3, the story of Abner reveals root issues to ailments of the stomach. Abner plays the role of a leader or teacher. There are a few twists and turns in the story that can be a bit challenging to follow but the stage is set for the unveiling of troubles with digestion, specifically the stomach. The stomach is the first location food enters after the mouth and throat, and if the stomach is not working properly food does not breakdown sufficiently, internal gases can become toxic and eventually result in numerous types of health disruptions

When the term King is used, it often refers to a powerful influence that rules over people. For many years people have fallen prey to powerful systems that have caused the human body to no longer have an ability to live in rhythm with the cosmic dance that is ever-present around earth's occupants. The earth has been subtly shifting its electro-magnetic, cosmic influence for the past few years. We are beginning to see some of this shifting in weather and season changes. People will need to make a shift as well, learning how to live with the rhythm of the magnetism they are becoming surrounded by. To live outside of this predicted and assigned "New Heaven and New Earth" atmosphere will place stress upon the physical body.

So, what could King David represent in the story? There could be multiple answers to that question but the most likely answer is, a powerful ruling situation (belief, lifestyle, item, etc.) over those who belong to God.

When the phrase "belong to God" or "child(ren) of God" is used in this publication, it is a reference to people who have a uniqueness to their genetic makeup or DNA. There is no label, to my knowledge, and thus "child of God" has been the identifier used. Something deep within the chemical structure of blood, DNA or even cells set a group of people apart from the remaining population. Scripture seems to blur references for this condition together through terms like Jew, Hebrew, Son, Child or Israelite. Aside from the ancient labels given, there is a unique identifier that remains to be discovered by science.

To keep the explanation short and somewhat understandable, cosmic signaling is required for the health of not only the brain but the body as a whole. When the brain is not capable of receiving the signals, the body will decline in health, the Heavenly Gases can become insufficient and "sin" sets in. An act of adultery (i.e., intimate attachment to anything outside of the natural order; crossing over into territory that is off-limits) as in the story of King David, represents the signal interruption, something that has come in and interrupts the healthy union between the human brain and the cosmic signals. (Territory that is off-limits according to the Laws of Nature can include: healthcare preferences, religious beliefs and practices, food selections, forms of exercise, clothing/fashion selections, etc.) Once this happens, generations that follow the initial incident can inherit a brain that is unable to receive the cosmic signaling required for health. The lack of proper signaling results in what this story calls a broken heart. The heart will not and cannot function at its intended capacity.

Before moving through the Chapters of this book, reading 2 Samuel Chapter 3, the story involving Abner, and Chapters 11 and 12, the story of King David and his act of adultery with Uriah's wife, Bathsheba, will be a benefit. It is within these stories that we will unlock the mysteries behind numerous health related issues experienced today. It is likely that somewhere along the lines of genealogy someone in the family has experienced the physical symptoms covered in this study. The keys to freedom from such things are just a heartbeat away!

Proverbs 3:1-2, 7-8

CHAPTER 1
LET'S BE CLEAR

Let's take a minute to address what "sin" is within the context of the story of King David. Sin is anything that disrupts the natural processes of the body or a person's lack of taking appropriate action (i.e., rebellion) to accommodate the body in its daily, weekly or monthly cycles required for health. Within the story of King David, you will notice two specifics about sin: 1) it will pass through genealogy; 2) it has a connection to the development or occurrence of a broken heart. As we know through witnessing the influence on the physical body when a heart attack occurs, a similar act occurs when the body no longer follows the commands of the cosmic activity, seasons and nature itself. Proverbs 20:9

Looking at spirit as being specific in its structural context, unseen, yet brings change, will help us unravel the message being relayed through the story of King David. Spirit is the term of choice used within Scripture to describe activity involving and often initiated by chemical elements. Chemical elements are around us every day, everywhere, and come from within the earth and throughout the Heavens.

Chemical reactions also occur through the foods we eat, creating gases that influence the function of the body. The specific combination of chemical elements that are beneficial to the body is what I call Heavenly Gases simply because at this point in time, there is no identified recipe for the measure and combination of gases necessary for the body to properly function.

Breath, air and wind are terms of choice used within Scripture to describe the movement of chemical elements and Heavenly Gases, their influence, how they can change things and that they are unseen. (Ezekiel 37:10; John 3:8)

The heart is the regulator for the Heavenly Gases within the physical body, pumping the gases that ride along with the plasma through the body. When the condition of the heart is hindered (broken), the gases that activate the various cleansing processes and provide energy in the body are not sufficient to maintain a healthy and disease-free body. We all know what takes place when the heart stops beating!

Now for the big one, rebellion. What exactly is rebellion? Rebellion encompasses acts that are contrary to a law or formal instruction, a strong resistance toward authority. Stubborn could fit in here as well.

1 Samuel 15:23
Job 34:37
Proverbs 17:11
2 Chronicles 10:19
Jeremiah 28:16

Space Activity

Laws are in place in the physical world as well as in the world of energy, electro-magnetic and chemical elements. The laws of what I call space activity, were put into place long before mankind, likely before and during creation. When the physical body is put in a position that runs contrary to the laws of space activity the physical body can and will eventually suffer in some way at some level. This suffering is a result of clashing with how the space activity works, how it flows or the momentum it has. Example: the law of gravity will not be in your favor if you jump off the top of a building. You will suffer a consequence, often referred to as a judgment in Scriptural text.

When interpreted correctly, many Scriptures in the Holy Bible describe how to conduct oneself in a manner that will benefit the physical life, assist in avoiding harm, and put a person in rhythm with the space activity. In this way, a person can live a more productive and longer, healthier life, avoiding death of the soul, and physical death by disease.

Out of Bounds

What causes this seemingly undetected heart condition? According to the story of King David the answer is rebellion that led to adultery, but adultery is not restricted to the physical act that would often come to mind. This adultery encompasses various acts that cause a person to become intimately involved with activities or lifestyles that are contrary to the space activity. (Proverbs 3:7-8) When a person participates in things contrary to space activity, the Star Dust (light; divine presence) is depleted. The activities that come to mind that people are routinely involved in are religious gatherings and exercise schedules (i.e., gym memberships).

Since the story at hand is from Scripture, I will use the example of religion, keeping in mind similar intimate connections occur in other forms. When a person becomes intimately involved with a religion, any of them, not just Christianity, to the point the person chooses the religion over what God established (space activity) or what nature dictates, that becomes adultery. The craving or mindset that puts the person in a position of feeling like they must attend and participate or "xyz" bad result will certainly happen to them. Is it the measure of excitement that comes from an adrenaline rush in response to a man-orchestrated event? What about the music, crowds and entertainment that cause a form of lust, that strong urge to be involved? That question has a multiple layered answer for now. No matter the recipe for the cause, people desire to satisfy the flesh. (Exodus 20:3-5)

A light-hearted example of an act of rebellion would be choosing to eat cheesecake or attend a ballgame on a Sabbath or New Moon Day when animal products should be avoided as a step in maintaining and achieving good health, and resting the body as prescribed for Sabbath to help the body recharge. This form of resting encompasses separation from crowds, noise, household chores and the job you may have during weekdays. Eventually the acts contrary to the Laws of Nature qualifies as rebellion. Most often the bigger issue is people are unaware that a violation is taking place. Mankind has become off-course and knowing or understanding how the very heartbeat of creation works was lost through time. Ignorance abounds! Hosea 4:6

People seem to have become mesmerized by daily or weekly gatherings where the idea is injected that attendance and/or money will bring a form of salvation (rescue). Ladies and Gentlemen, no one likes to be the messenger with bad news but, there is no salvation that brings a rescue from disease found within the walls of a religious organization or building, within an exercise routine or within a physician's prescribed treatment. To be rescued means to be removed from the disturbing or dangerous issue and brought to safety, no need for continual nursing the issue.

Nowhere in the creation story does it state that God created religion(s), vigorous exercise routines, events that involve large crowds and so forth. Many of these things were the idea of man and some just came into being due to the evolution of things. In Scripture, any gathering of a group of people was limited to certain days and times. Tribes lived amongst their own people and outside of that, people were isolated from one another.

Religions were formed by man and therefore contain a measure of error, no matter which religious circle you choose. Those errors have contributed to the downfall in human health because vital, life-giving information was erased from ancient instructions. The illustrations and storylines that have burped out through religions over time have developed into nothing more than regurgitated food particles. A big bunch of barf that now needs to be cleaned up! Religions are not alone as the medical professions are just as guilty. As long as the stories and studies continue to roll around as they have, the measure of sickness, disease, birth defects and so on will continue to rise. How or Why? The stories, illustrations and definitions produced through religions and other organizations are woven into the fibers of our being. When a person is exposed to a repetitive activity, like religious gatherings, exercise and so on, it becomes etched within the structure of the cells. Cells record sound, including words spoken, the environment that surrounds us, or simply posture and movement. Those cells pass through generations so whether a person has been involved in a religious circle (or other repetitive activity that falls outside of the commands) or not they can carry cells that have the religious recordings received from ancestors who did. Simply put, you inherit in your DNA the sermons, bible studies, marathons that were run, concerts attended or whatever it was.

Not every rule or idea inside a religious circle (or other repetitive activity) is authored by God. Mankind has contributed its share to the acceptable and unacceptable guidelines followed by many today. Things out of sync with how the body was designed to work on a cellular level creates a burden on the cellular rejuvenation process. Over time, the body can no longer fight off viruses or disease, balance necessary bacteria, and so on. The religious practices or exercise routine, etc. causes a burden for the body.

It would be wise to use caution when considering what God accepts or considers rebellious. The time has arrived for the Truth to come forth.

Doctor, Doctor

What about medical and dental care? There are times and cases when selecting a man-made drug or other form of manipulation over the natural processes the body will use to correct the situation becomes classified as adultery. Some forms of medical and dental intervention disrupt the ability to receive, process or house the Heavenly Gases required for daily physical function of the body and can deplete what I call Star Dust, light within the cells; the "divine presence" represented in the role of Uriah. Many dental procedures disrupt or even remove gases that the teeth attract and/or contain for function of the brain causing the intelligence level of the person to be compromised. Certain gases are required for the brain to work optimally and invasive dental procedures and even teeth whitening agents can disrupt what the brain requires for healthy function and intelligent thought processing. The teeth are powerful instruments.

To avoid an adultery situation in these matters, receive whatever medical or dental treatment is necessary for the time and then seek out a more natural alternative.

A person can easily become more comfortable with a man-made remedy, solution or quick-fix versus seeking answers through stillness, educating themselves on what is safe for the body, and listening for God's direction in the matter. America is focused on quick-fix remedies or solutions that are not always the best answer. The body is an amazing machine and when given the correct environment it will correct itself with proper time and attention. An education in the intricate details of how cells in the body work, the necessity of keeping the Heavenly Gases stable and in good proportion, and the seasons that keep them in rhythm is beneficial and, in some situations, required. There are situations when medical and/or dental intervention is absolutely necessary.

One Thing Leads to Another

Another good example is physical exercise. Medical professionals, along with many other avenues for healthcare, have taken the stance that "x" type of exercise that elevates the heart rate is required for health of the body. While I agree that a person should not live a sedentary life, I will also say that over-extending physical activity will deplete the Heavenly Gases the body needs to produce energy and keep the plasma clean. When you deplete the Heavenly Gases, the adrenal glands kick in and the result you have after the hour-long weightlifting, running, aerobic exercise, etc. is adrenal driven and eventually through time you will have adrenal fatigue. Adrenal fatigue can lead to a nervous system that is on over-drive. An adrenal system on over-drive can lead to insomnia. The body goes into survival mode and simply cannot relax. I have walked the adrenal fatigue road and can testify as to how miserable it can be. P.S. I do not recall any Scripture that indicates Jesus ran.

Aching and Breaking

Can a person die of a broken heart? Yes, a person can die of a broken heart although the process will likely be a long, drawn out one and come with a label other than broken heart.

Proverbs 16:3

Spirit and Heart Unite

Psalm 51:10-13

The verses in Psalm 51 shed light on the fact that there is a connection between the condition of the heart and the spirit. Again, Heavenly Gases/Spirit is the collection of specific chemical elements that the body requires for its proper function and daily energy. According to verse 10, the heart must be free (clean) of issues (sin) that create a hinderance for the body to receive and maintain a proper balance of Heavenly Gases. The physical body is a vehicle that operates through a means of gases (not gasoline) and electricity (brain and meridian activity). The "Holy Spirit," according to verse 11, cannot reside within or will be "taken away" from a body that has a broken heart. It is becoming evident that if there is disease in the body, there is sin, and the Holy Spirit cannot reside with sin. Those genetic imprints floating in the blood are what Scripture calls sin.

CHAPTER 2
THE BROKEN HEART

What qualifies as a broken heart? There are many things these days that can happen in a person's life that might result in an emotionally broken heart. Some common contributors to a broken heart one might see today would be physical or emotional trauma, verbal abuse, child abuse or molestation, guilt, loss of a relationship with a spouse, child or other close family member, and extended periods of grief. Could these emotional symptoms be a sign of a much deeper issue? One that involves the health of the heart organ itself?

The broken heart referenced in the story of King David can come through genetics, or it can be initiated by an individual's life experience. It is easy to identify the root of a broken heart when the initiating cause is experienced by the individual personally. What is challenging is to have genetic imprints from an ancestor who experienced a triggering event that trickles through generational lines and seemingly out of the blue a child that is quiet, passive, down in spirit, lacks happiness, exhibits low energy, has a chronic health condition, etc. is born. This makes the family wonder where the personality and physical condition of this child came from. Everyone else in the family is upbeat, chatty, outgoing and generally healthy.

Within the confines of the story of King David, a broken heart comes from rebellion, followed by adultery (stepping out of bounds), that then leads to murder and death (initiating a death sentence for others through genetics; loss of the light/divine presence). The act of selecting a lifestyle outside of the qualifying boundaries set forth in ancient text/Laws of Nature is rebellion that results in the broken heart. Herein could be an answer to chronic heart conditions. Ps. 51:1-3.

Why do I include adultery, murder and death as a cause for a broken heart? Because King David cries out for recovery from his contrite heart after he had 1) committed adultery with Bathsheba; (2 Samuel, Chapter 11); 2) arranged for the death of Bathsheba's husband, Uriah; and 3) death of his infant son. Adultery, murder and death are the center point of the story of King David.

Early stages of a broken heart can often be misinterpreted as depression, although clinical depression is not necessarily present. A broken heart can display as sadness, a lack of energy, being tired, lack of stamina which can then lead a person to experience the list of issues related to chemical imbalances that professionals identify as having gone astray. These chemical issues I'm referring to are things like adrenal fatigue, insufficient thyroid function, or hormone imbalance. These symptoms are all a result of the imbalance or lack of the Heavenly Gases, and the Heavenly Gases have become depleted in response to the broken heart. While various malfunctions in adrenal, thyroid or hormones may truly exist in a person experiencing a broken heart, it doesn't necessarily mean correcting or supporting the adrenals, thyroid or hormones will _rid_ the person of the root issue simply due to the root of the broken heart being embedded within the structure of the cells (personal experiences) or held within the structure of the DNA (inherited; Ps. 51:5). No matter the source, the broken heart must be addressed in order to avoid a lifetime of cyclical health issues, and a broken heart can be a challenge to change. Knowing where to begin is important.

Not every emotionally heartbreaking life situation will lead to a broken heart. The body is capable of processing and recovering its emotional balance when it is provided the correct tools. Stacking heartbreak upon heartbreak like one would see in a genetic situation is more challenging to overcome.

CHAPTER 3
FEAR VS. TRUST

Trusting and believing have been contaminated by a desire to understand. Harvest of Healing, LLC

Luke 21:26 KJV mentions men's hearts failing them in response to fear. What is fear? Lack of trust. It can be challenging to trust space activity mentioned earlier, or in the Laws of Nature, simply because people put their trust in evidence, and that evidence is often delivered through scientific studies or formulas. Nature does not work based on scientific studies. Nature works through chemical elements, magnetism and planet activity. It takes time to learn the signals and signs given by the Universe, the Sun, the Moon, the Stars, etc., but if people would take the time to give those things appropriate attention, stepping into rhythm with nature does not look or sound so odd, it just happens. Lack of trusting the natural order of things, or another way to say it is lack of trusting God, qualifies as fear. Live a life based on fear and a broken heart will surely ensue.

Too much knowledge causes us to miss out
on the conversation with wisdom.
Harvest of Healing, LLC

Proverbs 3:5-6: Trust in the Lord with all your heart and lean not on your own understanding; in all your ways acknowledge him and he shall direct your path. (NKJV) (emphasis added)

Proverbs 16:20

CHAPTER 4
VIOLATING THE OATH

2 Samuel 11:2-5

Bathsheba: Daughter (lineage) + seven (7=completeness, perfection, divine fulfillment). To take an oath.

Focusing on the "Bath" in Bathsheba brings about the concept of a bath, or being submerged, totally covered or engulfed by something is what comes to mind.

The descriptions of daughter and oath shed light on a spiritual issue (spirit activity is often represented in Scripture by a female), that comes along with a promise, the oath.

The number 7 reflects the day of rest. We are to work 6 days and rest on the 7th day. Currently, our 7th day falls on Saturday with Sunday being the beginning of the week, day 1. Day 7 is to be dedicated to providing rest for the physical body, not only in the form of relaxation and maybe a nap, but also for the digestive system. The rule I follow on day 7, known as Sabbath (there's that word bath again) in Scripture, is to remove leavening and animal products from my meals for that day. (For more on this subject see: Living by the Light of the Moon by Harvest of Healing, LLC published 2024)

With the acts of lust and adultery by King David, the picture painted within the story speaks of stepping out of a boundary set in place by an oath. The violation of the oath appears to have initiated an act of murder, meaning that the light or divine presence (Uriah) within the cells was removed and the position of sonship (death of the infant son) dies. The cleansing process that is brought about through the oath is violated and the physical body becomes contaminated with various debris.

The spiritual interpretation of the story of King David's adulterous act with Bathsheba has much deeper roots than the story often heard that gives instruction to avoid physical adultery. Adulterous acts against the spirit come with some serious health related consequences.

CHAPTER 5

DEATH OF URIAH

2 Samuel 11:14-27

Uriah: Light, flame or fire; divine presence, enlightenment or favor.

At this point in the story, as a result of King David's love affair with Bathsheba, David has a hidden agenda that sends Bathsheba's husband, Uriah, to the front of the battlefield lines. I would say King David was attempting to cover up his tracks and cause the public to think Bathsheba's pregnancy occurred during Uriah's brief return from the battlefield. King David's plan worked. Uriah ultimately loses his life in battle. According to this story in 2 Samuel, lust, adultery, murder, loss, and guilt all play a part in the development and progressive intensity of a broken heart.

The paragraph within the Introduction shares a few highlights on what the Husband figure represents in this story. As for Bathsheba, she is a representation of how the grass can appear greener on the other side, yet that "greener" grass will often result in severe consequences when a person steps beyond the boundaries set in place. This rule applies to things in nature, the things of God, and the way the Universe works. Follow the rules, Laws of Nature, seasons and so forth and things in life will move along fairly well. Step beyond the rules and things can get ugly. Uriah represents how the cosmic Husband connection is removed and dies through the acts taken that were outside of the set boundaries. When outside of the boundaries, the body will go through a physical battle in an attempt to survive.

CHAPTER 6

DEATH ON EVERY SIDE

Eliam: God + nation or people. God's people.
Nathan: To give; he gave; gift.

2 Samuel chapter 12 beginning in verse 1 is Nathan's parable delivered to King David. The parable describes a rich man and all that he has, and a poor, meek man and what little he has. This rich man, full of bounty on every side, takes from the poor man. The poor man is described as a traveler. Descriptions for traveler: moves from place-to-place; someone without a permanent home; someone who likes to vacation; or, in some circles it is a descriptive word for someone whose spirit through conscience travels during their sleep, a state of dreaming.

A Middle-English description from the 13th -15th Century defines "travailour" as someone who works hard or toils. The term is closely related to travail, which at that time meant laborious effort and travel. Whatever the case, to provide a better understanding of what is being said, I will interject some role-play here.

The rich man reflects a person who is fully in tune with the Laws of Nature, following the commands and laws with respect to seasons, moon cycles, food consumption, has an abundant supply, and so forth. Another way to say it is: The rich man is in sync with the Universe (God), and the Universe (God) treats him well. This rich man has an ample supply of resources for his life yet crosses a boundary and takes from or enjoys something that has little value. An act of toiling is involved with this item of lesser value. The poor man has a lamb, just one, not a herd. This poor man paid a price for this lamb. Lambs/sheep can represent innocence, but when considering Jesus, "the lamb who was slain," a lamb reflects a form of suffering to the point of death. The person who has it all in the form of good health, favor of God, worldly supply (rich man) goes to a source (poor man) and partakes of that source that leads to two death components. 1) death of the Husband connection; and 2) death of the sonship. The parable reveals that a lifestyle outside of the boundaries set in place will result in a price being paid that results in death.

When it comes to spirit-related consequences, or you could say energetic forces, there is a hierarchy, just like there can be in the physical. Referring to the built-in, God given qualities, when a person has all they need and more, it would be wise to stick with what is in their possession and not contaminate it by violating laws set in place thousands of years ago. When a person steps outside of the boundaries set forth by nature, fate, the Universe, select your preferred label, and take from or repeatedly enjoy something that is at a lesser rank than what you already possess, a form of death or erosion becomes attached to you. (See verses 5-6.) A similar concept would play out in a situation of a royal vs. a commoner. It's harder to bring a person up a rank than it is to take a person down a rank when you are dealing with blood components. A payment of four times the violation incurred will be required.

Bathsheba (oath) was the daughter of Eliam (God's people) and Bathsheba was violated by King David through the act of adultery (crossing a boundary; partaking of something that he was off limits). King David and his bloodline are now indebted four times the value of the violation. This makes for a hefty spirit/energetic force debt load. The payoff for these types of debts incurred will manifest in many forms. What initially comes to mind is costly health care or housing which could manifest into nursing care, general financial struggles, loss of a job due to health concerns, and so forth. What the initiating party does not pay toward this spirit/energetic debt prior to his/her death, will pass down to his/her heirs, and it keeps rolling downhill until the debt is paid. If a descendant adds to the debt, then the bloodline remains indebted for as many years and as many generations as it takes to get the debt fully paid. What happens in the physical realm also happens in the spirit realm.

There are commands that must be followed to avoid the death sentence described in verses 5-6. To despise the command(s) results in none other than the sword coming against you. Knowledge of those commands and how to apply them to life today is what is critical. Like many ancient teachings, the commands have lost their true definition and application.

2 Samuel Chapter 12, verses 9-10 warns that the "sword" will never leave the bloodline of King David. King David is reported to have despised (strong word) the commands of the Lord (natural law) and by doing so King David put a hefty consequence upon his bloodline. It appears King David was a rebellious type when it came to being in unison with how the natural order works. He thought the grass was more attractive on the other side where he was not allowed to be per the oath.

Swords are sharp, swift and deadly. This is a description of what death through disease will look like for those with a genetic imprint for a broken heart.

2 Samuel 12:11-14

As if the previous judgment was not hefty enough, the bloodline of King David will also experience separation from their wives. Today, this could be accomplished through divorce or death. It might be wise to think twice about casting a scowl toward someone who has been divorced, as the situation could be a consequence of fate, an "it is written" situation where the fingers should be pointed at King David who started the adultery ball rolling.

On a spiritual note, separation from a wife means the union with the cosmic Husband ends. As odd as it may sound, when the brain cannot receive signals from the moon or other planetary activity, the "spirit" within man is removed. Psalm 51:10-11

When a person in a position of power steps out of line with the laws etched in the very grain of the Universe, the consequences for the unlawful act taken will trickle down the bloodline. The King, President, Prince, Mayor, etc. does not only injure himself (or herself) but all those who are considered descendants and all who are under the rule of the guilty leader who has influence over the masses.

Likewise, as an example only: If a person lives a life in alignment with the rhythms of nature, has never been intimately involved with religion, never used prescription medications, etc., they can still have a genetic imprint for a broken heart when an ancestor who was, for example, a pastor of a church, or an active Buddhist or intimately involved in any other religion or organization that teaches contrary to the ancient laws etched in the Universe exists in their DNA. An avid exercise enthusiast or an ancestor who received an abundance of medical treatments can also create genetics for a broken heart. You may be innocent, but the ancestor(s) passed on the guilt of rebellion to you.

CHAPTER 7
LOSS OF SONSHIP

2 Samuel 12:15-23

In this portion of the story, Bathsheba's infant son dies. When actions are taken that result in a broken heart, like those connected to not following the commands, and the broken heart is not properly addressed, it can lead to the removal of the title of "Son" (offspring or heir) of God. The balance in Heavenly Gases (breath of God) is taken away and the connection to the cosmic signals (Husband) is gone. The person is no longer identified as having a position of "Son". Infant deaths (i.e., crib death) can be a sign of a genetic imprint for a broken heart.

Note the reference to fasting in verse 23. This verse indicates there is a form of recovery that includes fasting that will reestablish the Sonship position. (More on periodic fasting in Home-Made Answers for Cancer published 2024, by Harvest of Healing, LLC)

It is interesting to note that David spent the night lying on the ground (verse 16). Ground is a reference to a foundational or root issue. Loss of the status of son is a foundational issue when it comes to health. No "son," no "Husband" means the brain will eventually suffer and struggles in health will ignite. The reference to ground also directs attention to a flesh related issue. Soil = flesh.

Psalm 127:3
Romans 8:15, 23; 9:4
Galatians 4:5
Ephesians 1:5

CHAPTER 8

BIRTHING SOLOMON

Ammonite: Son of my people; beloved of Yahweh.
Jedidiah: God's friend; beloved or friend.
Joab: Yahweh is father; God is my father.
Rabbah: Great; many; abundant; great city.
Solomon: Peace, wholeness; man of peace.

2 Samuel 12:24-25

Things are looking up for King David and Bathsheba gives birth to Solomon. Nathan delivers a message to King David and Bathsheba, but Nathan refers to the child as Jedidiah, not Solomon. In these types of name reference situations combining the meaning of each name provides a deeper description, i.e. when a person is in a good relationship with "God" (space activity, chemical elements…) they will have peace. According to Jeremiah 8:11, mankind has been, and as of this date still is, separated from peace.

2 Samuel 12:26-31

There is a clash of forces between Joab and Rabbah who belonged to the Ammonites. The first 25 verses of Chapter 12 describe the downfall that takes place when a "child of God" (one who carries the Star Dust or specific DNA) steps outside of the commanded boundaries and death is a result. Good news, Joab, meaning Yahweh or God, gains the upper hand over the great city (meaning a collection of forces that stick together). In verse 27 there is a notation of the water supply. In previous publications information is shared about the water (plasma) in the body and how it can become full of debris. It is beginning to look as though stepping outside of the commands can lead to a health issue centered in the plasma.

King David comes along, after having lost his "son" (sonship) and is now in battle to regain the "Son" status by a means of recovering the crown (verse 30). In this portion of Scripture crown is referencing the crown of the head, an important meridian point used for receiving cosmic signals. Contaminated plasma can result in damage to the head/brain but according to the picture displayed through these verses, recovery from any damage done by dirty plasma can be had. It takes a battle between the forces, but it can be done. Two key elements used in regaining a healthy brain are 1) gold; 2) precious stone(s). The Scripture does not reference any particular stone. Personally, I rely on the stones used in the Priest's ephod. There are several stones that assist the brain in its normal function. A person does not necessarily have to wear the stones on their head, as in a crown. A piece of jewelry made of gold with precious stones set in it is sufficient, or simply placing a stone in the pocket of your clothing will do.

Solomon plays the role of achieving complete recovery from the broken heart. Temple construction does not take place until Solomon is in ruling position for four years. Once Solomon is in place for four years he (recovery) constructs the temple (the physical body; 1 Corinthians 6:19). There is a total of seven years from foundation to completion. This is the number of years it takes the physical body to eliminate "sin" and build new, healthy cells. Until people remove rebellion and *take the steps necessary to achieve recovery from the broken heart, peace will remain a lost item. Jeremiah 8:11). Once construction is complete, peace is achieved. The heart is clean and there is no more disease. It takes four years to reach the point of "construction" and additional years to achieve the full recovery resulting in peace.*

CHAPTER 9
LET'S NOT FORGET ABNER

Abishai: My father + gift or hope.
Abner: Father in a form of a community's alpha male, a social relationship + light or lamp. Father of light. (2 Samuel 3:17-39)
Asahel: To do or make + God; Healer or physician + divine presence.
Barabbas: Son of the father (yet a criminal).
Gibeon: Elevated place; place on a hill. (These descriptions can also be interpreted as arrogance or high-minded.)
Ishbosheth: Man or person + shame or disgrace.
Joab: Yahweh is Father; God has/is the fatherly role in terms of a social relationship.
Laish: Lion, a strong, lion-like figure; to knead, gentle.
Michal: Brook or stream; who is like God.
Paltiel: God is my deliverance; to escape; to bring into security.
Saul: Asked for; to ask.

Flipping back a few chapters to Chapter 3 of 2 Samuel we find the story of Abner. Given the meaning of Abner's name listed above, here is another story involving the loss of the internal light that has a little different twist to it. It appears that David has an on-again, off-again relationship with Abner as Abner continued to acquire power in the house of Saul.

The clash between Saul's "house" and David's "house" continues. The outline of the story of Saul and David has some similarities to the story of the crucifixion where Pilot gave the people the choice between Barabbas (Son of the father (teacher/leader), but a son who ends up being a criminal) and Jesus. The term house represents lifestyle, what is believed and how one lives.

Saul, a Benjamite, was the people's choice when it came to appointing a king. David (Judah) carried God's favor within and that favor gave David the upper hand in the conflict with Saul. Saul and David represent two powerful, influential spirit forces that have similar, yet different qualities. The flavor of jealousy began to taste good to Saul and he attempts to take David's life but fails. Saul ultimately takes his own life by falling on his sword. _Short interpretation here_: Powerful ruler selected by the masses will die by the means intended for use against its competitor. Saul could easily fit into the role of what scriptures call the thief that comes to steal, kill or destroy.

Women step into various scenes through the chapter. These women represent various spirit related activities that are intimate in nature (verse 6). Spirit forces begin to compete and clash with one another. This creates situations where accusations begin to fly!

In verse 8, Abner has become angry about accusations that originated from Ishbosheth (a person of shame, disgrace or confusion). The interesting part of the verse is where Abner states: "Am I a dog's head who belongs to Judah?" (HCS). This verse sounds a bit odd. What could it mean? Head is a reference to the mind, thoughts, logical thinking, or memory. It appears the text is referring to people who use logical thought processing when considering spiritual issues are called dogs. Domesticated dogs are often a reference to a person who is well trained to follow the commands of men.

In verse 10 it is revealed that there will be a transfer of power, leaving Saul's house and moving to David's house. David demands possession of Saul's daughter, Michal, (verse 14) and that possession transfer resulted in a separation of Michal from her current husband, Paltiel (God is my deliverance; to bring into security), son of Laish (gentle yet powerful). This separation from Paltiel is a picture of how Michal becomes separated from the cosmic Husband at the demand of something powerful (King).

By verse 17 it begins to appear that Abner plays the role of the middle-man, cordial to Saul's house and to David. Abner was appointed the role of bringing the people from the position of being Saul followers to being David followers. There seems to be a deception component on the part of Abner. He seems to be a bit of a spy. (verses 24-25).

Soon Abner is assassinated by Joab and his brother Abishai in the battle at Gibeon, piercing Abner in the stomach. Abner's death is noted to have been in revenge for the death of Asahel, Joab's brother. <u>Short interpretation</u>: Being deceptive, high-minded or arrogant removes the divine presence and will result in malfunction of the stomach.

Thus far, what is happening here in the story is a set of powerful forces clashing against each other that results in the internal light being removed from the region of the stomach. Seeking revenge, being deceptive, high-minded or arrogant (Gibeon) is where the death occurs. I do not interpret this revenge, deception, high-mindedness or arrogance as an individual issue although it can playout through individuals, but the root is present within a collective group or groups. The word battle tells us many people are involved at a large or wide-spread location that puts lives at risk. A root cause of stomach issues starts with revenge and deception that moves through high-minded, arrogant individuals or groups and results in a lack of internal light, and light is produced by the Heavenly Gases.

Verse 29 reveals a curse that ensues against Joab's house (leader/head of social gatherings). Judah's house of descendants is innocent of murder, but Joab's (social leaders/teachers) house of descendants encounters skin diseases, discharge, starvation, swift death and damage to chromosomes (in biology a spindle refers to the process of mitosis). Given the context of a curse, one can safely assume the reference to spindle points to some form of trouble with chromosomes during cell division. Herein could be an answer to Down Syndrome and other chromosome related disease or disability.

David realizes something bad has just taken place and he orders a time for mourning. (Verse 31). David is grief-stricken by the death of Abner and recites the following (verses 33 and 34):

Should Abner die as a fool dies? (interpretation: foolish choices will cause the light within to die out)

Your hands were not bound, your feet not placed in bronze shackles. (interpretation: freedom of choice)

You fell like one who falls victim to criminals. (interpretation: a relationship with unlawful acts will cause a person to fall to their death)

Verse 35 is where people came and encouraged David to eat bread while it was still day. Things become a little complex and interesting here. The verse states that David took an oath that states:

*"May God punish me and do so severely if I taste
bread or anything else before sunset!"*

*What is it about bread and hours of daylight? With the experience
I have had over the past six, nearly seven years, the only logical
explanation at this point would be the influence of hydrogen on the
body when the stomach is malfunctioning. Hydrogen is present in
wheat. When the physical body is without the internal light that
comes through the balanced Heavenly Gases, the hydrogen must have
a toxic or harmful reaction when eaten while the sun is at its highest
influence. The story indicates the light had died (Abner), the stomach
is in a state of malfunctioning and when fresh bread is eaten the
hydrogen could create a toxic gas response, resulting in what is called
a curse. If this is a possible scenario, there are many people today in
dire health situations simply by eating bread during daylight hours!
Although, I'm not sure how much of a hydrogen influence bread has
when it is mass produced and sits on shelves for weeks before being
consumed. Fresh bread is what would pack a punch if the stomach
were malfunctioning. How often is the function of the stomach
overlooked when various health issues arise, and professionals
are consulted? Remember, we are dealing with chemical elements,
the balance of Heavenly Gases. Something few, if any, health
professionals consider.*

At the end of the chapter, verse 39, David issues a powerful statement:

"May the Lord repay the evildoer according to his evil!"

*Ladies and Gentlemen, this story paints a clear picture of two
opposing, yet similar spirit forces. One creates life and one produces
death. On a strictly spiritual basis there are only two categories that
apply. Religions and the Laws of Nature. Religions are authored*

and run by man and can have some powerful areas of influence, but they can also result in physical ailments, illness, disease and death. To be blunt, death not only happens to the physical body, but the soul can also experience death prior to departing the body. No divine presence/internal light, no soul.

How does a person identify the dangers within the walls of organized religions? I'm not sure they are identifiable at this point, but watching for the signs is important. There are messages held within life events, such as the following:

I learned of some life events that took place amongst a small rural community of churchgoers that sparked my attention. This little country church had an attendance of maybe 30-35 locals each week. In the 1950s, during a stretch of a few months or maybe a year or two, the pastor of the country church died suddenly of a heart attack; one family lost an infant daughter to crib death; and the two-year-old of one family was struck in the face by a rattle snake and died. All these families attended the same country church, and all lived within a few miles of each other. No, not everyone is going to die of a stomach or heart issue. The point is when spirit forces (space activity) respond to certain human activities, words, motions, etc., to a point it shifts the electro-magnetic field in the atmosphere and becomes toxic or harmful, events such as the ones this small community experienced will unfold. It is the unseen electro-magnetic force that begins to influence our surroundings, our bodies, animals, and so forth. Until the initiating and damaging forms of spirit forces/space activity are identified, it might be wise to close the doors, let things air out for a while and simply stay home. There is a benefit in letting the dust settle so observations are clearer, and awareness is had. Once the harmful initiating events can be identified, gathering will take on a new appearance and the occurrence of life-threatening situations will wane. For now, we do not know what the changes will encompass.

An important component to the demise within religious gatherings is rigid structure to the weekly services. What am I referencing here? Each week Sunday School begins at 10:00 a.m. with church service to follow at 11:00 a.m. or, people enter the church, curtsy and kneel, sing a song and listen to a priest or pastor speak. We must not forget the time of "praise and worship". News flash here, praise and worship have nothing to do with singing a song while various instruments create their noise. That's a concert. Praise generates from within, and worship is reverence. All of these church related activities seem harmless, right? At least two things are at play here. Children are to receive instruction up to a specific age. Once that age is reached, the child, now teen or young adult, is to have a measure of ability to step out on their own. The lessons have been seeded and have begun to grow so the responsibility is now upon the shoulders of the young adult with the watchful eye of a parent or leader. Adults are to be mature and responsible for their life, receiving little instruction outside of their own Scripture study and at an advanced mature age, they retire from their life duties connected to teaching or mentoring. This type of structure flows with nature. It appears that anything outside of this pattern of instruction is simply a social gathering hidden within the label called glorified in some way.

Religious communities also need to be become aware of and honor seasons. The different seasons bring about different lessons and positions for a person. Like the New Moon does not fall on the exact same day of the week or calendar date and moves with the ebbs and flows of spirit force, so shall we be. Lessons respective of this pattern seem to have been tossed out the window. There is much to be learned and at this point it is obvious no one person knows how the service of the church is to be run to be in sync with the Laws. What we do know is continual stirring of the current pot of soup is causing havoc.

The Holy Bible scriptures and many ancient texts that existed before the writing and publication of it were instructions for obtaining and maintaining good health. The Holy Bible was not intended to be a religious manual. Taking instruction that was put into place for the specific reason of guiding one through health-related obstacles and putting it into a different context is classified as gossip. A dab here and there may have a taste of truth, but the majority of it is folly. Herein is where humanity has walked their way into trouble and the judgments for such actions continue to pour out.

On the HarvestofHealing.com website there is an article called Rapture Inside the Four Walls posted May 9, 2025, that will shed more light upon the issues. It may be well worth the time to read that article.

CHAPTER 10

HOUSEKEEPING

The Heavenly Gases (Spirit) are the cleaning crew for the physical body as they ride along through the veins by means of the plasma, clearing out debris from the various tissues and organs in the body. When a broken heart is present and the Heavenly Gases within the body lack the ability to remain in proper balance and provide good health, how does a person go about gaining ground in recovery? The broken heart needs the gases to heal, and the gases need the heart to maintain balance and distribution. The very source needed for recovery of the broken heart is hindered by the broken heart itself. (Ps. 51:11) A vicious cycle is in place and attempting to "think" your way out of it does not work.

Once a broken heart has taken root, the electrical signals it gives off become embedded in the cells. Being embedded in the cells creates a situation of repeated bouts of the sadness, feeling tired or down, lack of strength, and many other symptoms. Now the person has a cyclical set of symptoms that truly cannot be changed by "thinking differently," participating in counseling or support groups, meditation, caffeine, or any other relief mechanism of choice. While the participation in any one of various therapies may bring a level of temporary relief, they will not and cannot change the reoccurrence of the record held within the cells. Therapies can help a person to manage a reoccurring symptom or memory, but they cannot rid the body of what is recorded within a cell. In these cases, one must find what works to relieve the intolerable situation that runs its cycle every "x" days, weeks or months until a clean heart is evident. The condition of the heart is at the root of the symptoms experienced.

Eliminating a lifestyle that runs contrary to the Laws of Nature is a good form of housekeeping.

CHAPTER 11

CHRIST BRINGS
THE CLEAN HEART

If King David cried out for his heart to become "clean," you could say healed of the burden of sin, then there is a way to overcome this heart ailment that does not include a long list of various therapies, drugs or supplements. Therapies we know today did not exist in the days of King David and remedies for ailing health or injuries consisted of any combination of herbs and oils, precious metals and gemstones.

Christ is the term used in Scripture to refer to a process that takes place in the blood, achieved through living within the commands. Those commands include consumption of food, hygiene, clothing, sleeping arrangements and so on.

Blood of a fetus, then to infant and on to child lacks purification simply because of the various infections and toxins the parents were exposed to prior to conceiving a child. (Ps. 51:5) There is a process that is required once a person is at or beyond a specified age to cleanse the blood of genetically inherited contamination, commonly called genetic mutations, and self-encountered contaminates. I am hopeful that future generations will be born with contaminate-free genetics and clean plasma and blood.

Phase 2 of the cleansing process is to <u>maintain</u> the purified blood achieved. This maintenance involves the living by the Laws of Nature with respect to what Scripture calls Sabbath (resting the physical body, inside and out), how we are to respect specific phases of the Moon, the application of herbs, oils, precious metals and gemstones, what, how and when we eat, and so on.

The proper measure of Heavenly Gases, coupled with time, patience and strict obedience to Sabbath and Moon phase laws results in the blood becoming clean of debris (sin) and a status of Christ is birthed. I go into the detail of this process in prior publications.

Proverbs 20:9
Psalm 24:4

CHAPTER 12
A DOSE OF HUMILITY

Psalm 51 is King David's cry for restoration. The reality of "Oops I screwed up" kicked in and King David humbled himself, crying out to God in a petition for help. King David admits the mess that he had created could only be cleaned up by God's natural order, not through a doctor or therapy session. Verse 17 mentions a humble heart. Humility was the first step to freedom.

To be humble does not mean letting people or situations run you over. To be humble means to recognize the authority that exists and adhere to it rather than traveling the road of what is popular or what man says is good or right. Not everything posted on the internet or broadcast over soundwaves is beneficial for everyone. Yes, there are laws on earth that we must follow but there are also choices that can be made.

Being humble and respecting what the spirit can perform on the interior and exterior of the physical body is a critical piece in the recovery from a broken heart. A person must be willing to allow the simple, yet complex Laws of Nature take their course. This does not mean sitting and doing nothing. It means attention will be directed most often to remedies and forms of relief that are contrary to what popular opinion or even scientific studies have to say.

With humility comes repentance in the form of changing what is being done. Lifestyles and choices must change, leaving the toxic, harmful lifestyle behind and stepping into rhythm with the commands set forth that bring abundant life to the physical body and the soul.

Psalm 4:7-8
John 10:10

CHAPTER 13

SACRED DINING

Chapter 12 states that King David would not eat "with them". There are strict rules about who a son (aka the righteous) should eat with or amongst. When a meal is eaten with individuals who do not follow the mealtime rules and food regulations assigned by nature and held within the orchestration of their blood, a debit type of action takes place against the soul (the life/light spoken of earlier). Eating in a restaurant is a good example of eating with strangers. The righteous person's soul can be debited for every unrighteous person's act of eating what is considered unclean. Yikes. This might make one think twice about eating with large groups, particularly with strangers or those who have values different or unknown to you. Similar to the system of banking, too many debits can result in bankruptcy.

The food a person chooses to consume plays a role in the balance or imbalance of Heavenly Gases within the body. Another zinger to this topic is blood chemistry. Think of a chemistry lab. When mixing foods and liquids together in any number of arrangements, chemical reactions will result, good or bad. Could these chemical reactions involving foods be an answer to how different blood types are now present? The diet of many Americans and other ethnic groups has blown good health to pieces.

A person's blood chemistry will determine the influence any one food will have on the production of Heavenly Gases and functionality of the systems and cycles the body requires. When it comes to influencing a person's health, there are certainly many food combinations and choices involved. Selecting what is most beneficial, and considering genetics is what is critical. It would be wise to observe how nature works (when to eat, what to eat, portions, weather/seasons) and ask God (Universe, Source) for guidance. Feeling well or energized is not always a reliable gauge for how healthy a physical body is when it comes to functioning through/with the Heavenly Gases.

It can be a challenging feat to change, rearrange or eliminate certain eating habits. I know this to be true. Once the initial stages of cravings and habitual hunger pangs are past, the changes come easier and relief to the body will begin to be had. It takes determination and patience.

Ezekiel 34:10

CHAPTER 14

ESSENTIAL OILS

Psalm 51:7 mentions Hyssop for purification. The essential oil Hyssop can be used topically or defused. When using topically, it is advised to dilute the oil in a carrier oil such as jojoba or coconut.

Essential oils are potent and therefore, a little dab will do. Likely just a drop or two.

CHAPTER 15

A RESULT OF PRAISE

Moving through the remainder of Chapter 51 in Psalms, we see that praise will come forth from the body by means of the tongue, lips and mouth. This praise is not through verbally singing a song. This praise is from the inside of the body and connects to the breath (inhale/exhale of gases), evidence of a cleanliness within the body. The physical body of humans and animals were made as instruments for balancing the electro-magnetic fields that we live in. If there was not an instrument for balancing those fields, the force within and surrounding the earth would be too great for man and animal to survive on its surface. Praise is a form of achieving and then honoring what has been instituted by God, the Universe, the Source and nature.

People must learn to dance in rhythm with nature, to be in step with its every shift and change. Observe wildlife to gain some knowledge on how this is done. This dance with nature is guided through the use of color, gemstones, clothing fashion, food selections, lifestyle choices and so on. Details for the dance have been previously published and written by Harvest of Healing, LLC. (Eating Yourself to Death, Chapter 1, God is the Galaxy; and The Powerful Influence of Clothing: Color, Fashion, Style)

The following lines may resonate with some:

Praise God from whom all blessings flow.
Praise Him all creatures here below.
Praise Him above the Heavenly Hosts.
Praise God, Father, Son and Holy Ghost.

The second verse describes it all:

Praise God the Father who is the source.
Praise God the Son who is the course.
Praise God the Spirit who is the flow.
Praise God our portion here below.

Praise: the expression of approval; admiration.

Psalm 30:5; 150:6
Jeremiah 20:13

CHAPTER 16

WHAT HAVE WE DONE?

At the onset of creation certain soundwaves and vibrations were put into place. The electro-magnetism of the earth was at its best. As time progressed and population numbers increased, the birth of motorized machines, technology and satellite beams moved in. Systems were established, religious beliefs branched off into various directions and disturbance in the Heavenlies began. Temperature fluctuations, tropical storms, drought and tornadoes became common occurrences. What have we done?

Tension in the atmosphere builds, animals become aggressive, frightened of their human neighbors. Insects increase in population and kind, unidentified bacteria appear, and viruses are discovered. What have we done?

As stories are told behind the walls used for social gatherings and labeled as religious meetings began to take on a new meaning, becoming amplified through various sound systems, human words of altered truth were raised to the Heavens, clashing with the existing natural order established during creation. The clash of nature vs. religion echoes throughout the atmosphere, depositing its residue amongst people and animals. Chaos abounds and peace has escaped. Time was shattered, seasonal shifts were changed from one calendar month to another, and the ability for humans and animals to live in harmony and connect with the Heavens ceased. Calendared months and Holidays can no longer be calculated as they once were two thousand years ago simply due to the cosmic shift. People are now celebrating historical events out of time. The chaos increases. The love affair with the world changed everything. Like lambs being led to slaughter, so are we. What have we done?

For peace to return, altered stories and contaminated words must cease to proceed from the mouth. (Proverbs 18:21) Whether those words come through music, curse words, general conversation, or church sermons, the cosmos responds to the corruption, no matter the source. It is time to reconsider what is being spoken. What have we done?

For the sake of mankind, the animal kingdom and the earth, it would be wise to lay all disruptive things aside and wait for peace to reign on the earth once again.

May the atmosphere of the Garden of Eden prior to corruption once again be established. In the Name of Jesus.

CONCLUSION

BLIND TRUST

Trust does not always come with a clear road map
Many curves are set before you that can feel like a trap.

Put one foot in front of the other as you go
Before you know it, life moves with the flow.

Trusting can be a challenge when you cannot see
The results you expect in response to your plea.

What you expect may be different than what you receive
Remain steadfast and in the end you will see
That trust pays off and you will be free.

No more sorrow, guilt or shame
All because of an ability to trust in His name.

Harvest of Healing, LLC

Izauh 61®

RESOURCES

Holy Bible:
Holman Christian Standard
New King James Version

Suggested Reading:
From AntiChrist to I AM
Food for the Journey to I AM
      Published 2022, Harvest of Healing, LLC

Home-Made Answers for Cancer and Life Altering Disease
      Published 2024, Harvest of Healing, LLC
Living by the Light of the Moon
      Published 2024, Harvest of Healing, LLC
Eating Yourself to Death
      Published 2024, Harvest of Healing, LLC
The Powerful Influence of Clothing: Color, Fabric, Style
      Published 2025, Harvest of Healing, LLC